NutriFitUp 7-day Detox

Iulia Bledea
Mother,

Devoted Wife,
Ambitious Fitness Coach,
Nutritionist Technician

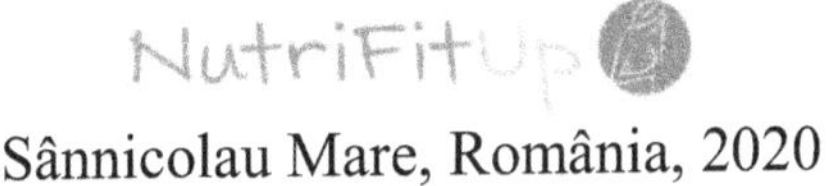

Sânnicolau Mare, România, 2020

Contact us:
NutriFitUp
contact@nutrifitup.com
www.nutrifitup.com

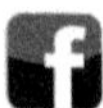   @NutriFitUp

   @NutriFitUp

The National Library of Romania CIP Description
BLEDEA, IULIA
   NutriFitUp 7 - day Detox / Iulia Bledea.... - Sânnicolau Mare :
Nutrifitup, 2020
   Contents bibliography
   ISBN 978-606-95001-5-6

613

Special thanks to:
         Desktop publishing:
         Prof. Cornelia Catrina
         Mecatrin: tehnoredactare.mecatrin.ro

Cover Design:

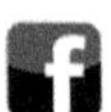   Papur Project – Ioana Stirbu

Photo Design:

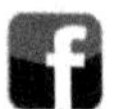   Papur Project – Ioana Stirbu
         Miriam Silas – photos

Project manager:

   George Balaniuc: ***Dream, apply, repeat!***

Contents

The following work, entirely or partly, is under copyright protection according to Law no 8/1996 regarding copyright and related rights.

NutriFit-Up SRL, the copyright owner of this work, mentions the following aspects for their readers:

★ **According to art. 140 of Law no. 8/1996, the reproduction of the works or products under copyright protection or other related rights without the copyright owner's authorization or consent constitutes an offense and it is punished with imprisonment from one month to a year or with fine;**

★ **According to art. 14 of Law no.8/1996, by reproduction, within the meaning of the present law, shall be understood the making of one or more copies of a work, in any material form, the making of any audiovisual recording of a work inclusive, as well as its permanent or temporary storage by electronic means.**

★ **According to art. 196, distributing a work without the consent of the owner is punished with imprisonment from one month to a year or with fine.**

NutriFitUp SRL has the right to act, through law and involvement of authorities when it comes to civil, administrative and criminal liability regarding the persons who reproduce a work or distribute it to unauthorized parties, including on sharing channels, uploading in internet groups, share via e-mail or other communication channels, making physical copies or distributing them to authorized parties.

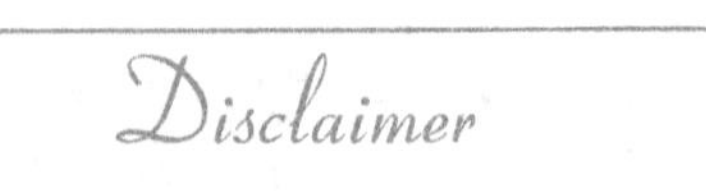

Disclaimer

NutriFitUp S.R.L. products are not meant to diagnose, treat, cure or prevent diseases.

Any information provided by this book and/or by other products are not meant, under any circumstances, to replace the specialized medical advice, diagnosis or treatment.

The information available in this book has a general characteristic. NutriFitUp S.R.L., its employees, partners and/or associates do not take responsibility for the accuracy and correctness of the information presented.

NutriFitUp S.R.L., its employees, partners and/or associates do not take responsibility for any occurring health incidents or damages.

We always encourage you to talk to your doctor about the information related to your treatment or medical condition.

> **Warning!**
> Psyllium husk is very healthy, but one should bear in mind that people who are prone to constipation, irritable bowel syndrome and other symptoms, might have mild flatulence and prolonged constipation throughout the detox, in which case they should seek their doctor's advice.

★ This detox might contain allergens: gluten, lactose.

★ If you are allergic to any of the ingredients, replace that ingredient with another one from the following day's menu or from another one's which you like best; or replace that particular meal with one from another day. (For example, lunch from Day 1 can be replaced with the one from Day 3).

★ *NutriFitUp S.R.L. and its associates do not take any risk which might be implied from you reading this book.*

Why is detox important?

It cleanses your colon. Detox offers you more chances to lose weight, as it helps treating problems which prevent you from losing weight. It regulates inflammation and reduces digestive problems.

Detox is wonderful for the blood sugar levels.

It is a process which leads to a physical and emotional release. It is a period during which you can put on hold your hectic lifestyle. You can combine detox with relaxing baths, yoga or meditation. Another good idea would be to journal your moods as well.

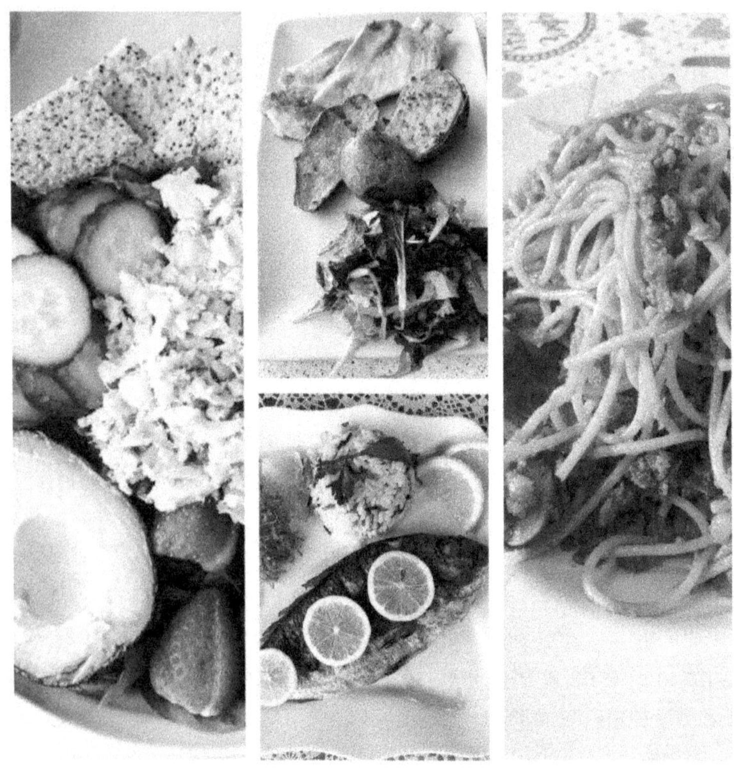

Introduction

Hello!

I am Iulia Bledea, cofounder of NutriFitUp, mother of two magnificent daughters, who bring me joy and smiles every day, a devoted wife, nutritionist technician and ambitious Fitness Trainer.

I study continuously and I love everything related to sport, nutrition and, with the help of my own techniques developed in time, I managed to change the lives of many people, some of them in a quite advanced state of obesity.

I have been practicing different sports for over 10 years (swimming, gymnastics, handball, tennis, aerobics, fitness), and I have gained knowledge, experience and training methods so that you can enjoy the best results.

If you were to ask me, I would say the biggest experience I gained was during my two pregnancies, and when I became the mother of my two absolutely gorgeous girls. Knowing that food plays an important part in my children's health, I had to pay even more attention to this aspect.

I have been through gaining and losing weight twice, reaching my ideal weight, hence I do have experience and I definitely can help you lose weight, shed those extra kilos.

I am still studying and I think that if I stop, I will become very dull. Out of this work satisfaction came an even bigger desire, that is, to help millions of women lose weight.

NutriFitUp recommendations and guidelines

READ THE BOOK, THE ENTIRE BOOK.

Check the questions, and then, if you do not understand something or have any questions, search it in the NutriFitUp VIP group, and, if you still do not find it, post it on the GROUP!

I do live sessions weekly and answer questions!

Thank you for understanding!

FAQs:

1. Am I allowed to drink coffee?

   ◊ **Yes**, you are allowed to, after your meal. You can add stevia or coconut sugar. Coffee is drank after meals, but not more than 200 ml, milk included, as it is enough.

2. Can I drink or have a snack between meals?

   ◊ **No**. You fast or drink just water between meals. Your stomach need breaks, so does the whole digestive, hormonal system.

1. What do I do if I can't find an ingredient?

   ◊ You replace it. A fruit, with another fruit, a vegetable with another one, and meat with another type of meat.

   NOT TO BE REPLACED: BRAN AND FLAXSEED.

1. Where can I find the products featured in the book?

   ◊ In apothecary shops, supermarkets, natural products websites. You can find more details regarding the source of the products on our group.

1. I need to drink more water than indicated, can I do that?

   ◊ Always listen to your body, **of course you can**!

6. I can't eat everything, I can't drink all the water, what do I do?

   ◊ My dear, have a little patience, don't force yourself into eating everything, eat the whole meal step by step, drink the water gradually, until you reach the recommended amount.

7. I work in shifts, how do I do this?

   ◊ You are not alone, here's the solution: It doesn't matter if you work 1st, 2nd or 3rd shift, you prepare the meal that comes next and, during the work breaks you eat it; when you sleep, you sleep, and when you wake up, you eat the next meal.

1. I don't like an ingredient, what do I do?

   ◊ Try eating it, change comes in small steps, use spices to make the transition easier.

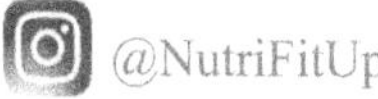

9. I simply can't, drinking bran or seeds makes me nauseous, what do I do?

    ◊   Add lemon juice and drink a small amount gradually. If you give up, it makes no sense saying you detoxed.

10. I can't drink lemon water.

    ◊   You'll learn to like it. If you have no medical restrictions, drink lemon water daily, it helps with the permanent detox process.

11. I fast, what do I do?

    ◊   70 g quinoa – replaces meat.
    ◊   150 g mushrooms – replaces meat.
    ◊   100 g tofu – replaces cow cheese.
    ◊   200 ml almond milk – replaces a snack
    ◊   One soy yogurt – replaces cheese or yogurt.

12. Do I eat whole flaxseed or ground flaxseed?

    ◊   **WHOLE FLAXSEED.** Their role here is different.

13. I don't like mashed peas or creamy soup, what can I do?

    ◊   All I can recommend is help your body cleanse. It is your choice if you want to follow my advice or not. These foods are necessary, if you don't eat them, you can't say you did a right detox.

14. Do I weight the food raw or cooked?

    ◊   Always raw. ☺

15. When can I start exercising?

   ◊　Throughout the whole detox, whether you run, walk, whether you choose to do the exercises in the book or not. Exercising is important!

16. What color should lentils be?

   ◊　It does not matter. It is a healthy product I recommend regardless of its color.

17. Can I drink alcohol during the detox?

   ◊　**No**. Now is not the time to drink. After the detox, you can occasionally drink a glass of wine.

18. Can my husband do this detox?

   ◊　Yes, but snacks have to be doubled. For example, an apple will become 2 apples, 20 g of peanuts will become 40 g. **The minimum water intake for men is of 2,5 liters !**

What is this book? 

This book is a "break" for your stomach and brain, a restart, and, why not, a new food approach.

I am sure you will find this new information useful!

Thanks to detox, sport and healthy food, women have managed to lose weight, love themselves, accept themselves and feel good in their own skin.

You must definitely accept yourself as you are, but you have the right to wish for a change. In order to lose weight, this detox will be the start for your dream look.

I know you want to be skinny, to change your clothes' size, I know all about these wishes, because there was a time when I had the same feelings and I managed to fulfill my wishes. As a result, I invite you to go through the book, READ IT, and then get to work.

You won't fail, as what you will experience applying this detox worked for so many women, that I managed to change not only the lifestyle, but also the thoughts from "I can't" to "I did it!"

Why is it important to have a LONGTERM healthy lifestyle?

Body detox is an ongoing process, which has to be maintained throughout the WHOLE life.

This little guide is a small example of what you should eat in order to have a carefree life.

If you won't establish the bases of a healthy life through exercising, a balanced diet and positive thinking, you have chosen the 7 Days Detox in vain.

Detox is a regenerating process which you need to do!

Over 5,202 women on the NutriFitUp VIP group made it.

What do you choose?

How can you tell you need a detox?

I congratulate you on the decision taken to read and apply this detox and I assure you are on the right path. I invite you to take this road to wellbeing together, towards more health, vitality and a dream body!

★ Do you feel out of sorts?

★ Do you feel like you need more rest and wish to stay in bed longer?

★ Headaches?

★ Bloating?

★ Skin rashes?

★ Constipation?

Processed foods are bad for your body!

Please make a list of all the products you frequently eat, then read their label and you'll surely be amazed by the high quantity of food additives, those allowed preservatives which do not harm if consumed rarely and in small quantities, but in the long run and high amounts, can lead to intoxication and the slowing down of your metabolism.

You will find a list of all these additives at the end of this book, so you can see the harmless and the harmful ones.

E-numbers, body disorders such as: overloading the liver and pancreas, and when these organs cannot function properly anymore, where do all the unhealthy residue go? In the colon! Are you familiar with the notions of colon cancer, multiple sclerosis, ulcer?

Sugar intake can cause metabolism disorders, mental disorders as well as cancer.

Allow me to let you in on all the bad consequences of E numbers' frequent consumption and I guarantee you'll be surprised about how well you'll feel if you stop eating them.

Food additives are made through synthesis that affects all the cells in time, influencing the leukocyte formula. Their role is to preserve, color or, in the worst case, give foods a fake taste.

Producers consider using additives because they are cheaper and stronger compared to their natural counterparts, and my recommendation as a mother and nutritionist technician is for you and your family to avoid eating foods that contain additives.

Since they can be found almost in all foods, you will ask me: "Then what am I supposed to eat?"

On the secret group NutriFitUp VIP, I post daily menus, recipes and natural foods, their source, as I am always looking for those products which do not have additives or have been the least affected by them.

Join our NutriFitUp VIP group to find out as many useful pieces of information for you and your family.

How does this detox work?

This detox will give you a boost of energy because the main ingredients used to maintain the body in detox are 100% natural!

We use three main ingredients: **psyllium bran, wheat bran** and **flaxseed.**

By consuming the recommended fibers daily, you will help your body cleanse itself so that you'll be able to notice a beneficial change in your body.

Let me introduce you to the benefits of these ingredients on the body, namely:

★ **Psyllium**: it reduces sugar and fat absorption, thus controlling weight.

It increases the feeling of fullness while adding the minimum amount of calories. The fibers in the psyllium bran have a high capacity to absorb water, so that they grow in your stomach and quickly make you feel full. They contribute to controlling blood sugar levels, reducing the postprandial glycemic response, being recommended as a treatment for obesity and diabetes.

It is very recommended in all detox diets, as it reduces the sugar and fat absorption.

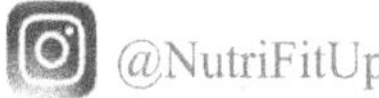

Properties:

Psyllium bran contains 14 less soluble fiber than oatmeal, which was much appreciated until lately, for its high content of fibers. 100 g of psyllium contain approximately 71 grams of soluble bran, while for the same amount of oatmeal there are only 5 g of soluble fiber.

★ **Flaxseed**: it is used to stimulate metabolism. This type of seeds help in treating intestinal inflammation. It can be cultivated anywhere, countries with hot climates.

Properties:

Due to the high amount of Omega 3 fats, the flaxseed has an emollient and lubricating effect on the colon, thus favoring the elimination of hardened feces which stay for days in the colon of people who suffer from constipation.

★ **Wheat bran**: this is practically the outer shell of the wheat, which is often thrown away.

Properties:

Wheat bran is a natural fortifier, which helps to improve digestion and refreshes the body through nutrients, with no contraindications or notable side effects. Due to its proven remineralising, antimicrobial and anti-inflammatory properties, having a diet based on wheat bran for a month or two is a natural solution for health problems such as anemia, physical and mental fatigue, constipation, phlebitis and thrombophlebitis, cholelithiasis and colitis.

In order to begin a new lifestyle, you need a detox, a restart, a new beginning. It's just like moving into a new house.

What do you do when you move into a new house? You clean up, right? That's why detox is important, it comes as a restart and gets the body ready for what comes next, that is, a new lifestyle. This is the basic principle I apply when working with women who want a slim silhouette but also a healthy lifestyle.

There are people who refuse this detox and, of course, they end up wasting time, stagnating on the same results and making the progress slow. The intestinal walls are stuffed with toxins, gastric acid is on high levels, the bile's activity is hardened by unhealthy food, alcohol, smoking and excessive medicine.

★　**Ioana, an active member: "I can't, it's too much for me!"**

Currently, Ioana is exercising 5 times a week, has been practising the breathing technique which you'll find in this book and, of course, she has changed her mindset.

From "I can't" she has come to say: "I want, I can!" Ioana was obese, and because of this she was dealing with depression and she entered a vicious circle, she would constantly eat chocolate, which satisfied her cravings, so her body would give off endorphins and serotonin, but she did not eat properly, made her liver and stomach tired and her acidity increased.

Where am I going with this? If you don't say STOP to unhealthy habits on time, they will lead you, you will feel disappointed, you'll end up having depression. Due to the excessive use of unhealthy foods, your metabolism will grow "old" and calories burns will be hampered because of the unhealthy food you give your body, thinking you are doing well.

Having ties with the beauty and body care areas as well, I have met many women who were self-conscious, lacking self-confidence, because they were weighing more than the idea standard, they had a tummy and they were getting tired easily.

Some of them were realizing it, saying that they need to do something, while others were finding excuses saying "I have been pregnant", "I take after my father/mother", "I don't have time", "It is hard", etc.

Napoleon Hill used to say:

"The mind knows no other boundaries than the ones we set ourselves."

I am not absurd, nor do I want to criticize your lifestyle, but if your body sends off signals, I think it is time to listen to them and make a change. High cholesterol, diabetes, high blood pressure, cellulite, visceral fat (see the explanation in the dictionary), spots, constipation, diarrhea, all these are early signs of a stroke or a heart attack.

Studies show that people who eat processed foods, trans fats, drink alcohol or smoke are more prone to a heart attack, diabetic coma, high cholesterol, high blood pressure or cancer. Blood flow through blood vessels is made difficult and the blood loses its quality.

I also taste "forbidden foods," but I know what to do afterwards.

What is intestinal barrier or gut health?

Let me explain...

An optimal level of health is the answer to a proper functioning of the intestinal barrier or the mucosal layer. How does it deteriorate? The intestine with a high permeability, defined medically as the permeable bowel syndrome, is characterized by boosting the permeability of the intestinal lining for a number of endogenous and exogenous toxins.

Endogenous toxins are produced by the body and the exogenous ones are produced through indigestion.

This disorder comes up when the spaces between the intestinal wall have widened, for various reasons, and they allow toxins to come into the body. The intestine loses its protection, due to the intake of: refined sugar (white), unknown refined foods, low intake of vegetable fibers (precisely what I have written above), using antibiotics, poor digestion, Zinc deficit, alcohol abuse, anti-inflammatory abuse (aspirin, ibuprofen, etc), stress, sadness, anger. Inflammations occur as a result of a misled lifestyle, smoking and alcohol.

The food that we eat affects each function, whether we like it or not.

If we eat unhealthy food more often, we will start feeling its negative effects in a few years. Remember! Not now but in a few years.

But what happens if you eat healthy? It's easy! You are full of energy and feel like a different person!

The signs of a traumatized or permeable intestine are: allergies, anxiety, headaches, rashes, low immune system, bloating, diarrhea or constipation, fatigue (see the images below).

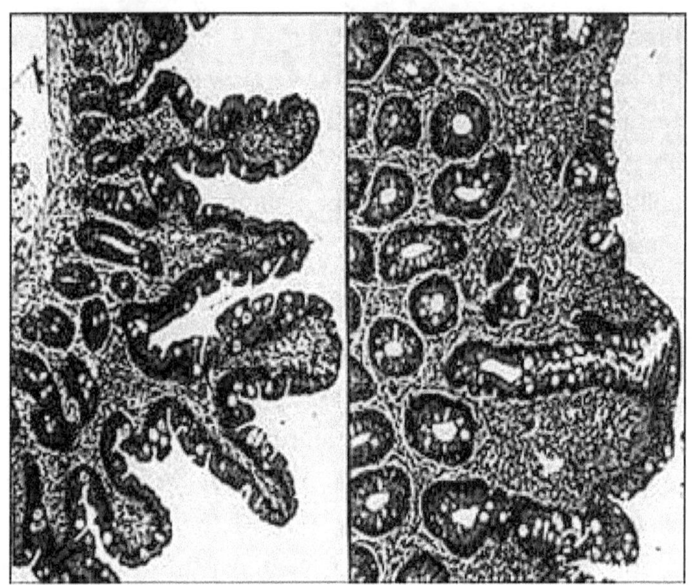

In the left image we can see the intestine with the clean villi, functioning at high parameters, and on the right, the villi are literally blocked by toxins and other residue, as well as being inflamed.

Hence the constipation and disorders presented earlier.

IMPORTANT:
NutriFitUp Recommendations

Detox might not always be pleasant, but its beneficial effect on the body and the relief feeling will make any sacrifice worth it, as this slow detox prepares you for a new lifestyle.

Detox can be done for 7 up to 10 days. For the rest of the days, just pick any menu from the other days,
you can just do that! ☺

For chronic constipation, you should eat psyllium bran in water every morning, for 10 days in a row, following this process every month until the constipation symptoms have been removed.

For people with bloating or constipation problems I recommend, even after finishing detox, drinking a glass of water with psyllium bran every morning for a month, or repeating this detox 5-6 times a year.

SPORT IS NOT A WHIM. IT'S NOT SOMETHING YOU WEAR TODAY AND GOES OUT OF FASHION TOMORROW.

SPORT IS MY FAVORITE ACCESSORY!

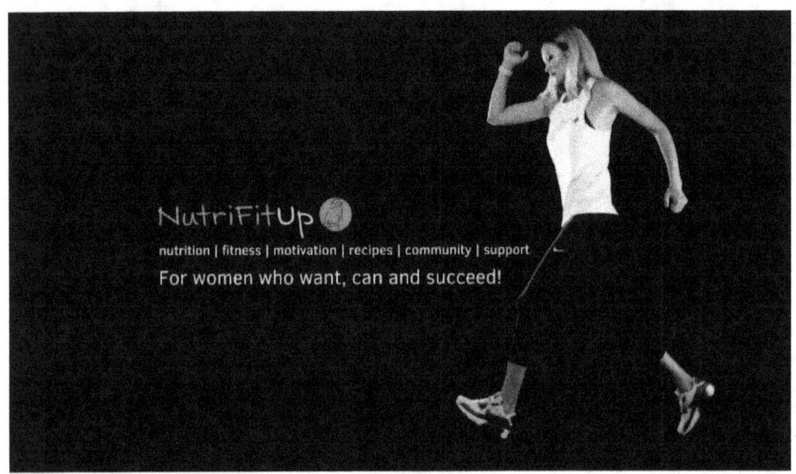

Chapter 1
Detox - The first step towards your goals!

Why is it so important?

◊   It cleanses the digestive tract;

◊   It treats chronic constipation;

◊   It prevents and treats diarrhea;

◊   It prevents colon cancer, the toxic substances being absorbed by it;

◊   It reduces the level of bad cholesterol;

◊   Contributes to weight control;

◊   Reduces bloating;

Detox purifies the body, but you should also consider purifying your soul. What does that mean? It has been proven that there is a connection between feelings, emotions and the physical state.

Get rid of the stress which causes hyperacidity (detox the body and change your body and soul), get rid of negative thoughts (forgive, love, and accept what you cannot change!), spend time with your family, love and cherish yourself. Start the day by meditating 5 minutes! Say "Thank you!" to the One above and... think differently!

Detox is recommended for all categories of people: obese, smokers, sedentary people, and even people with no problems. In order to start a new lifestyle, a nutritional plan or a change, a detox is mandatory. Otherwise, we risk eating healthy and yet no results may turn up because of the toxins gathered on the intestine, fats on the liver, bile ducts, lazy bile or other problems.

For this detox you will need some ingredients that can be found in any apothecary shops, and some products to ease digestion. You will notice limiting carbs for this detox. This does not imply giving up carbs completely, just throughout the detox period.

If you have chronic or acute problems I advise you not to consume carbs (rice, potatoes, pasta) alongside with meat, because the digestion time is different and in some cases it may cause bloating.

Nevertheless, I recommend complex carbs such as whole grain brown rice or pasta. They have no gluten and they are very healthy.

You will find the list of ingredients attached and thus you will be able to easily buy what you need (you can take a picture and look on your phone, it's more practical; or you could cut it with scissors and take it with you).

Detox is divided into 7 days. You will do it during this period, and then you can follow it again after 2-3 months. This is a gentle diet, it does not attack digestion, it does not irritate the stomach lining, all its ingredients are natural.

HELP! CONSTIPATION!

How can you fight this unpleasant problem?

Most people have dealt with this unpleasant situation at least once in their lives.

First of all, it is very important to know the cause. You can find this out through a medical examination, to make sure it's not a genetic problem.

However, if it is due to not paying attention to meals and the quality of food, then you could easily apply our advice.

Constipation occurs when there are insufficient fibers, liquids or an imbalanced diet.

It can be a sign of excessive calcium or iron intake.

Low thyroid hormone could also produce constipation in most cases.

For me, the most unpleasant aspect is not going to the toilet daily.

Constipation can cause a certain skin odor, halitosis or coated tongue.

Blocking the transit stops eliminating toxins from the body, so a regular intestinal transit will get you rid of your toxins!

Solution?

Constipation can be prevented, treated and of course, you can get rid of it.

☞ Exercise daily for at least 30 minutes, using the Training Book.

☞ Include more fibers into your diet daily.

☞ Essential acids (found in flaxseed)

☞ Eat spirulina or chlorella

☞ Eat friendly bacteria from yogurt such as sana, kefir.

☞ INSTEAD OF THE RECOMMENDED BREAKFAST EAT 2 spoons of natural prune jam, 150 ml of water, 1 spoon of psyllium bran, 1 orange.

☞ Drink more water! (Check your necessary daily water intake by using the formula 0.04 l water*your weight in kilograms).

Drink water 30 minutes before eating to stimulate digestion.

☞ **I recommend starting a weight loss diet immediately after detox.**

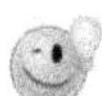 **Please write down the kg you have now, how many cm for your waist and tummy...**

For example:

★ If you have chosen the 7-day and you start on Monday, you will weigh yourself the following Monday.

★ If you have chosen 10-day detox and you start on Monday, then you will weigh yourself the following Thursday.

★ Members of the group wanted to take before and after pictures, and so can you, if you want, for a more satisfactory documentation.

Date	Kilograms before starting Detox (waist and tummy cm)	Kilograms after finishing the 7-10 day detox (waist and tummy cm)	If you feel excellent after the detox, draw a heart here. Congratulations!

For a faster progress, I advise you to start your day with positive affirmations: "I want, I can, I know, I can do it!". Exercise daily for at least 30 minutes to fight off the sedentary lifestyle.

Another thing I advise you to do properly: learn how to breathe correctly!

What does that mean? Is your first thought in the morning related to work, money or stress? Maybe you sigh, maybe you don't bring your brain the optimum level of oxygen, so that your thoughts are clouded and so is your whole blood flow.

The first thought we should all wake up with is gratitude! We live under the impression that we are entitled to everything, but we often forget to be grateful to the Divinity for simply existing!

Breathe in holding the air for 10 seconds and your diaphragm extended, and breathe out decompressing the diaphragm until you eliminate the whole air.

Repeat this process daily! It takes only one minute of your time!

Motivation

> **Be the change you want to see in others!**
>
> *Trying to change the world before changing ourselves means swimming against the stream. No outside change can occur if there is no change on the inside. As within, so without.*
>
> *Neville Goddard*

Why did I choose this quote? To make you understand that if you persuade your mind to do one thing, your body will follow. If you start off the wrong foot and say you can't, this is exactly what will happen. It is the law of attraction, what you think shall happen.

If you truly want something, you will make time. And you will make it! If you are positive and optimistic, you will surely surpass any situation. If you are pessimistic it is time to apply all things stated above. And stop being like that... it's not good for you.

Detox your body and your mindset. Start the day with energy and positive vibes: So what if it's Monday? So what if it rains? If will rain some more, it will be Monday again, what is important is how you enjoy the rain... you can sit inside all grumpy or you can dance in the rain.

> **"There are only two choices: you either progress, or you make excuses and lose."**

How can you educate yourself on food nutrition?

Read the labels! You can't eat something unless you know what it contains! Learn to educate yourself and be a responsible woman, a mother who puts only the right food on the table!

Start to playfully introduce the basic food principles to your children.

I recommended some foods, but it's within your power to check the producers.

You won't live your life with rules and diets, so make your life easier by choosing tasty, nice looking ingredients!

Chapter 2:

Shopping list and the 7 days of detox

👆 **IMPORTANT:** if you think the products are too expensive for your budget, choose more days in a row to consume the certain foods, but you must eat the bran and seeds every day!

★ 1 bag of wheat bran (200 g)

★ 1 bag of psyllium bran (200 g)

★ 1 bag of flaxseed, pumpkin seeds (50-100 g)

★ 5 lemons, rocket, baby spinach

★ 1 bag of frozen peas, lentils, red beans (100-200 g)

★ 1 bag of baby carrots (200 g) broccoli, raw almonds (100 g), apple, kiwi, orange, pomegranate

★ 1 pack of fresh or frozen blueberries

★ 2-3 sana, kefir, yogurt (200 ml) or natural yogurt 2-3% fat (150-200 g)

★ Turkey breast, chamomile tea, marigold tea (1 bag)

★ Chicken breast, green onion, whole grain rye bread

★ Water 10 l (still), 1 can of tuna (120-150 g)

★ yogurt 2% fat (120-150 g) – if you chose the ones that you find in a store (I recommend you join the VIP group to find out which is the best)

★ Goat or cow milk – If you choose to make your own yogurt

★ Oats, nuts

★ Almond milk, Kalamata olives, extravirgin olive oil

★ Grapefruit, cucumber, goji (50 g)

★ Chia seeds (100 g), 3 eggs.

★ Chicken, pig or cow bones (make sure they are from a safe source)

Day 1

7:00 – 8:00 eat a spoon of psyllium bran mixed with 150 ml of water on an empty stomach.

Eat right away.

If you find it hard to drink, mix it with half of a squeezed orange, lemon juice and/or natural apple juice.

If you let it sit for a few minutes, you will notice a gel will form. This gel has beneficial effects on your stomach lining, that is why it is important to drink the bran right away.

After 15 minutes, drink another big glass of warm water (300 ml) with lemon (half a lemon squeezed). It has a laxative effect and it cleans the digestive tract.

I recommend you to wait for an hour after drinking the bran, and then you can have:

★ Breakfast

Almond milk oats

🕐 Timeline: 08:00-09:00

How to prepare:

2 spoons of oats in 150 ml of almond milk, 10 g of goji and a teaspoon of chia seeds (placed in a bowl of water the night before and consumed in the morning).

Calories: **350 kcal**

Properties of oats:

They are gluten free, and excellent source of fibers, proteins, minerals. They are excellent in choosing a healthy breakfast.

Contraindications:

Like any other healthy ingredient, if consumed excessively, it can cause some unpleasant reactions. There are no studies to say that oats can cause diseases or imbalances. It contains a toxin called which is not dangerous for human health.

🥛 Drink water after 30 minutes.

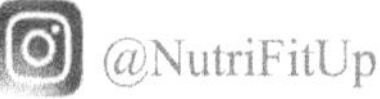

★ Snack 1

Red grapefruit

🕐 Time: 11:00

★ Eat your red grapefruit snack.

Calories: 100 g - 35 kcal

Properties:

It contains insoluble fibers called pectins, which protect the stomach lining and regulate cholesterol, they instill the fullness sensation due to a high quantity of fibers.

Nutritional composition:

100 g grapefruit have 30 – 35 kcal, 0, 65 g protein, 0, 1 lipids, 8, 08 carbs, 6-7 sugars, calcium, magnesium, iron, phosphorus, potassium, zinc, vitamin C, folic acid, vitamin A.

Contraindications:

There are no studies to certify this, because we can talk about a problem when there is an excessive amount of fruit consumed. People with biliary disorders have experienced unpleasant sensations when consuming this fruit. If you are one of them, eat an orange instead.

Drink water after 30 minutes.

★ Lunch

Carrot and pea mash with chicken breast

🕐 Timeline: 13:00 – 14:00:

★ 100 g of pea mash or boiled peas, 100 g of carrot mash and 150 g of grilled chicken breast.

Calories: **450 kcal**

How to prepare:

Spice the chicken breast, grill it or boil it; boil the carrots until they become slightly soft – do not boil it for too much time, or else it loses its nutritional value. Put them in a blender, mix, add salt and pepper, a spoon of light yogurt and a little bit of mint for taste and flavor.

Boil the peas for 10 minutes, blend it, add a spoon of yogurt, salt, pepper, a little bit of chili, a clove of garlic and mix them together.

Properties:

Antioxidants, anti-inflammatory, fights against gastric cancer and reduces the risk of diabetes. Peas contain: vitamins A,B,C,K, phosphorus, magnesium, zinc, selenium, and carrots contain vitamins B1, B2, B6, A, C, E, K, P, Pp, a remedy in detox and certain diseases.

Contraindications:

It is not recommended for people who suffer from kidney stones.

🥛 Drink water after 30 minutes.

★ Snack 2

Kefir with wheat bran

🕐　Time 16:00 – 17:00

★　kefir yogurt 200 ml and a teaspoon of wheat bran.

Calories: **120 kcal**

Properties:

This snack is high in vitamin E, calcium and has a high amount of fibers and iron.

Bran contain vitamins (betacarotene, B1, B2, B3, B5, B6, B8, B9, E), amino-acids, carbs and minerals.

Yogurt is rich in calcium.

🥛　Drink water after 30 minutes.

🥛　Drink two more glasses until dinner!

☝　**Hydrate the flaxseed in water!**

★ Dinner

Salad

🕐 Timeline: 19:00 – 20:00

★ Eat a 300 g salad, made up of rocket, baby spinach, a spoon of boiled lentils, a spoon or boiled red beans, a teaspoon of pumpkin seeds, a spoon of flaxseed (hydrated in water for 2 hours) and 100 g of yogurt.

Calories: **450 kcal**

How to prepare:

Put all the ingredients in a ceramic or glass bowl, mix them, add salt and add some lemon juice. You can add chopped parsley and a spoon of extra virgin olive oil.

Properties:

Rich in fatty acids, sterols, stanols, fibers, chlorophyll and vitamin K. It helps lower the bad cholesterol, and provides the necessary fibers and vitamins.

Contraindications:

None.

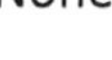
Drink 200 ml of water after an hour.

Drink a glass of water with a teaspoon of flaxseed before bed.

Day 2

🥛 07:00 – 08:00: Start the day with a glass of water and a spoon of psyllium bran, and a teaspoon of flaxseed hydrated in water for 4-5 hours.

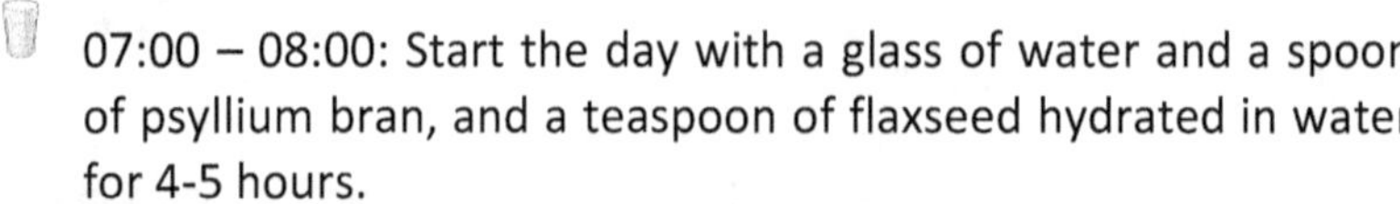

Put the seed in water overnight, and the bran in the morning.

🥛 Drink a glass of warm lemon water after 15 minutes.

★ Breakfast

Fruit salad

🕐 Timeline: 08:00-09:00

An apple, a kiwi, an orange and half a pomegranate with 50 g chia, 100 ml of water.

Calories: **450 kcal.**

How to prepare:

Mix everything together in a blender or smoothie maker.

Properties:

Fruits are an excellent source of vitamin, energy and they contain vitamins such as vitamin C, B, K and minerals such as iron and magnesium.

Contraindications:

None

🥛 Drink marigold tea (200 ml) after an hour because it has a strong disinfectant role.

★ Snack 1

Blueberry yogurt

🕐　11:00

A plain yogurt with 2 spoons of blueberries

Calories: **140 kcal.**

Properties:

Yogurt is an important source of calcium and proteins, especially casein; blueberries contain amino-acids, antioxidants such as vitamins A, C, E and K.

Contraindications:

None!

🥛　Drink water after 30 minutes.

★ Lunch

Turkey breast with vegetables

🕐 Timeline: 13:00-14:00:

150 g turkey breast, 100 g broccoli and 100 g green beans.

Calories: **450 kcal**

How to prepare:

Cook in the oven or steam. Vegetables get cooked faster, so do not cook them along with the meat, you add them 20 minutes before the meat is ready. Spice the meat with garlic, salt, pepper, coriander, and let sit a few hours before cooking.

Properties:

Broccoli and green beans are rich in chlorophyll, they contain vitamin K, C, E. Meat is a high source of proteins, amino-acids and vitamins.

Contraindications:

People with thyroid disorders will take into consideration the doctor's recommendations.

🥛 Drink approximately 300 ml of water after 30 minutes.

★ Snack 2

Walnuts and yogurt

🕐　16:00 - 17:00

20 g walnuts, hydrated in yogurt for an hour.

Calories: **140 kcal.**

Properties:

Walnuts contain selenium, they lower triglycerides, they are a strong source of antioxidants, fat omega 3 acids, arginine, fibers and minerals.

Contraindications:

In big quantities, it can cause constipation. That is why it is important to consider each product's quantity for this detox.

Drink water after 30 minutes.

Drink water before dinner!

★ Dinner

Lentils with egg white, cucumber and olives

🕐　Timeline: 19:00 - 20:00:

2 spoons of lentils, 3 boiled egg whites, a cucumber, 10 olives.

Calories: **400 kcal.**

How to prepare:

Boil the eggs, separate the yolk, add the boiled lentils, cucumbers and olives. You can mix them all together like a salad, or put them separately on a plate.

Properties:

Lentils are a good source of plant protein high in selenium and manganese. Egg white contains albumin and proteins. Pepper contains vitamin A, betacarotene and is low in calories, ideal for losing weight and detox. Olives contain vitamin E, calcium and iron.

Contraindications:

None.

🥛　Drink water afterwards.

🥛　Before bed: drink 1 glass of water with a teaspoon of flaxseed hydrated in water for about 4-5 hours.

Day 3

Start the day with a spoon of wheat bran mixed with 200 ml of warm water.

REMEMBER! Add lemon or orange juice if it is too hard to drink. Drink right away!

After 15 minutes drink a big glass of unsweetened marigold tea (strong disinfectant).

Boil a delicious and nutritious broth: bone broth with vegetables. It sounds weird, but the nutritional value is superior to any other meal.

You need: 5 bones with a little meat, one carrot, one celery, 1 pepper, 1 onion, 1 teaspoon of salt.

How to prepare:

If you have a multi-cooker, put all the ingredients together and let boil for 12 hours.

If you do not have this machine which makes your work and life easier, let everything simmer for 5-6 hours. Put water just to cover the bones.

You can eat the broth with your family, it has collagen, protein and repairs the stomach lining.

This soup can replace a meal. You choose when to eat this soup, preferably at dinner.

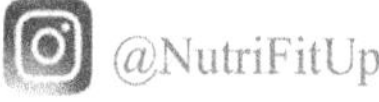

★ Breakfast

Bread with yogurt and flaxseed

🕐　Timeline: 08:00-09:00

2 wholemeal rye bread slices, chemical free, with a yogurt with two teaspoons of seeds. Add dill and salt on the toast.

Calories: **400 kcal**

How to prepare:

Toast the bread, add dill and some chives on top, it will improve the taste.

Properties:

Wholemeal bread is a source of energy as it is considered a complex carb, recognised by the body, unlike the white flour refined bread, which is not good for eating, as it causes an imbalance in the colon, destroying the lining.

Contraindications:

None!

🥛　Drink a mug of marigold tea after an hour.

★ Snack 1

One grapefruit

🕐 11:00

One grapefruit.

Calories: **100 g - 35 kcal**

Properties:

It is beneficial, as it helps eliminate the adipose tissue. Rich in fibers, nutrients and antioxidants, it supports the proper functioning of the body.

Contraindications:

None!

🥛 Drink water after 30 minutes.

🥛 Drink a glass of water and hour before your meal.

★ Lunch

Tuna salad

🕐 Timeline: 13:00 - 14:00.

Tuna salad: 120 g tuna, 150 g lettuce. Choose the tuna carefully, make sure it is in chunks and in water.

Calories: **450 kcal**

How to prepare

Spice the lettuce with salt, pepper, lemon, dried tomatoes and add the tuna.

Properties:

Tuna is rich in vitamin E, it has Omega 3, 6, 9. Lettuce has vitamin K and vitamin C.

Contraindications:

None.

🥛 Drink water after an hour.

★ Snack 2

Almond milk

🕐　Timeline: 16:00-17:00

A glass of almond milk – 200 ml

Calories: **160 kcal**

Properties:
Low in calories, it gives you energy!

Contraindications:
None!

After an hour, drink some chamomile tea, it helps reduce bloating.

★ Dinner

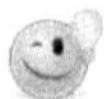 **Chicken breast with grilled vegetables**

🕐 Timeline: 19:00 – 20:00:

Chicken breast with grilled vegetables: 150 g chicken breast and 100 g vegetables.

Calories: **450 kcal**

How to prepare:

Spice the chicken with salt, pepper and a little garlic, and grill until it is golden. You can choose a frozen vegetable mix or fresh vegetables from the garden/market.

You will use 100 g of vegetables. Grill them, spray some lemon juice, add some rosemary and a spoon of olive oil at the end.

Properties:

This dinner contains proteins, fibers and vitamins from the B complex. It is a light meal, suitable for anyone.

Contraindications:

None!

🥛 Drink water after 30 minutes.

🥛 Drink a 200 ml glass of water and a spoon of psyllium bran, and drink another one after 15 minutes.

Shopping list for the last days:

- ★ Raisins, avocado
- ★ Apple
- ★ Broccoli
- ★ Pear
- ★ Kohlrabi
- ★ Beetroot
- ★ 4 carrots
- ★ Celery
- ★ Grapefruit
- ★ Sesame seeds
- ★ Trout
- ★ Mango
- ★ Tomato paste
- ★ Chicken/beef liver
- ★ Olives
- ★ Cucumber
- ★ Orange
- ★ Sweet potatoes
- ★ Linden tea
- ★ Basil
- ★ Rosemary
- ★ Green beans
- ★ Turkey leg
- ★ Raw pumpkin seeds
- ★ Banana
- ★ Raw almonds
- ★ Barley flakes
- ★ Oat flakes
- ★ Red beans (ifyou have some left, do not buy some more)
- ★ Chickpeas
- ★ Light Mozzarella
- ★ Forest fruits
- ★ Coconut
- ★ Brussel sprouts
- ★ Coconut milk
- ★ 3 Cucumbers
- ★ Red onion
- ★ Pistachio
- ★ Cauliflower
- ★ Cinnamon
- ★ Cheese
- ★ Parsley
- ★ Parsnip
- ★ 3 eggs, almond milk

Day 4

07:00-08:00 as soon as you wake up, drink a glass of water with a spoon of wheat bran, add some lemon juice too.

After 15 minutes, drink 200 ml of marigold tea – don't forget its disinfectant effect.

★ Breakfast

Almond milk oats

Timeline: 08:00-09:00

150 ml almond milk, 50 g oats, a spoon of coconut flakes and 5 raisins.

Calories: **400 kcal**

How to prepare:

Mix all the ingredients in a blender.

Properties:

Oats contain beta-glucan fibers, known as superfoods, as they cleanse the intestine, reduce cholesterol and repair the lining of the intestinal walls.

Contraindications:

None.

Drink water after 30 minutes.

Drink a glass of water after lunch.

★ Snack 1

An apple

🕐 11:00

A big apple.
Calories: **100 kcal**

Properties:

Apples contain fibers called pectines, which help keeping the whole digestive system healthy, reduce inflammation and support immunity!

Contraindications:

None!

Drink water after 30 minutes.

Drink a glass of water before your meal.

★ Lunch

Cream of broccoli soup

🕐 Timeline: 13:00 -14:00

Cream of broccoli soup
Calories: **400 kcal**

How to prepare:

Boil 300 g broccoli in salted water; when it is slightly soft, take it out, blend it, add a light yogurt with a spoon of olive oil, a garlic clove, salt, pepper, parsley leaves or allspice; serve with a slice of wholemeal toast.

Properties:

Broccoli, as a green vegetable, is a great source of vitamin K, rich in vitamin C, A, and the B vitamin complex.

Contraindications:

None.

🥛 Drink a big cup of marigold tea after an hour.

★ Snack 2

Pistachio

🕑　Timeline: 16:00-17:00:

20 g raw pistachio .
Calories: **100 kcal**

Properties:

Excellent source of essential fatty acids, calcium, iron and potassium. It reduces the level of bad cholesterol, boosting the good cholesterol!

Contraindications:

None.

🥛　Drink a glass of water before dinner.

★ Dinner

Salad

🕐　Timeline: 19:00 – 20:00:

Salad.
Calories: **450 kcal**

How to prepare:

Grate a kohlrabi, a beetroot, a carrot, half a celery and a ripe avocado. Add olive oil, sesame seeds, salt and pepper.

Properties:

It contains tocopherols, vitamin A, E, K, betacarotene, sodium, potassium. It is the most impressive salad, as it combines many flavors.

Contraindications:

None!

- Drink a glass of water an hour after eating dinner.

- Drink a glass of water and a spoon of flaxseed (hydrated in water 4-5 hours before).

- Don't forget to prepare the pudding in the evening, so you can eat it in the morning!

Day 5

- 07:00-08:00: start this day with a 200 ml glass of warm water and a spoon of psyllium bran.
- Drink 200 ml of linden tea 15 minutes after.

★ Breakfast

Chia pudding

- Timeline: 09:00-10:00

Chia pudding, hydrated in almond the night before and 2 spoons of fruit.
Calories: **400 kcal**

How to prepare:

90 ml almond milk and 40 g of chia seeds, a spoon of forest fruits or a freshly cut fruit (you can add the other mango half you are going to use for the next day snack). Mix these ingredients at night and let sit in the fridge in a covered glass bowl.

Properties:

It contains 3 times more proteins than meat, iron, calcium and lots of fibers! It is an excellent combination when talking about a dessert!

Contraindications:

None!

- Drink water after an hour!

★ Snack 1

Mango

🕐 Time 11:00:

100 g mango.
Calories: **120 kcal**

Properties:

It is rich in vitamin C, antioxidants, and vitamin K.

Contraindications:

None!

Drink water after an hour!

Drink a glass of water before lunch.

★ Snack 1

★ Lunch

Cauliflower with Brussels sprouts and chicken/beef liver

🕐 Timeline: 13:00 – 14:00

150 g of roasted cauliflower, 100 g Brussels sprouts or cabbage and 100 g of chicken/beef liver
Calories: **400 kcal**

How to prepare:

Put half a mug of water in a pan, boil the liver, and cover it with a lid. Add a chopped red onion, 2 garlic cloves and a spoon of homemade tomato sauce or just a plain tomato paste. Boil everything for 15 minutes. Put the cauliflower in the oven, then eat it along with the liver.

Properties:

Cauliflowers contain anti-cancer phytochemicals, stanols and phenols. Liver is an important source of vitamin A.

Contraindications:

None.

🥛 After an hour, drink linden tea with lemon and a teaspoon of honey.

★ Snack 2

Pistachio

🕐 Timeline: 16:00 – 17:00

20 g raw pistachio
Calories: **120 kcal**

Properties:

Important source of essential fatty acids. It supports the nervous system.

Contraindications:

None.

🥛 Drink water after an hour!

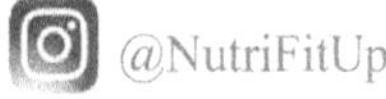

★ Dinner

Greek salad

🕐　Timeline: 19:00-20:00:

Greek salad: 5 black olives, a chopped tomato, 1 cucumber, ½ red onion, 100 g of light cow, sheep or goat milk cheese.
Calories: **450 kcal**

How to prepare:

Chop all the ingredients and add a spoon of olive oil and basil.

Properties:

It contains iron, proteins and essencial fatty acids.

Contraindications:

None!

🥛　Drink water after an hour!

🥛　Drink a glass of water with flaxseed previously hydrated in water for at least 3-4 hours.

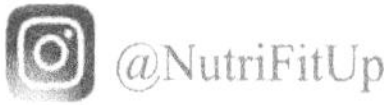

Day 6

You're almost there!

- 07:00 - 08:00: water with wheat bran, 200 ml water and a spoon of bran

- Drink 200 ml after 15 minutes.

★ Breakfast

Boiled eggs with cucumber

🕐 Timeline: 08:00-09:00:

Two boiled eggs, one cucumber and a wholemeal slice of toast.
Calories: **400 kcal**

Properties:

It contains proteins, albumin, betacarotene and vitamins C and B.

Contraindications:

Egg (especially the yolk) can cause allergies in some cases.

- Drink water after 30 minutes.

★ Snack 1

An orange

🕐　Ora 11:00:

An orange
Calories: **120 kcal**

Properties:

It contains vitamin C, fibers and sugars. Is supports immunity and the digestive system.

Contraindications:

None!

Drink 200 ml of water after an hour.

★ Lunch

Sweet potatoes with trout

🕐　Timeline: 13:00 - 14:00:

100 g sweet potatoes with 150 g trout baked in the oven
Calories: **450 kcal**

How to prepare:

Spice the trout with rosemary, Himalayan salt, 2 slices of lemon and put in the oven for 20-25 minutes next to the potatoes.

Properties:

It contains manganese, potassium, iron, calcium and proteins, being a meal rich in vitamins. Sweet potatoes are healthier than the white ones. They contain vitamin E, Omega 3, 6, and 9, which help lower the bad cholesterol.

Contraindications:

None

🥤　Drink 200 ml of water after an hour.

★ Snack 2

Pumpkin seeds

🕑 Ora 16:00:

15 g of raw pumpkin seeds hydrated in water for an hour.
Calories: **100 kcal**

Properties:

Helps intestinal lining. They contain manganese, iron, copper, zinc and antioxidants.

Contraindications:

None.

🥛 Drink water of tea after an hour.

★ Dinner

Green beans with turkey leg

🕐 Timeline: 19:00 – 20:00

200 g green beans boiled or roasted, 150 g of turkey leg.
Calories: **400 kcal**

☝ **Prepare the lunch for tomorrow!**

How to prepare:

Spice the turkey leg, place in the oven and when it is almost ready, add the green beans.

Properties:

It contains vitamin K, potassium and vitamins from the B complex. Meat is a very important source of iron and proteins.

Contraindications:

None!

🥛 Drink water after an hour.

🥛 Before bed, drink a glass of water with a teaspoon of flaxseed, previously hydrated for about 4-5 hours.

Day 7

Last day!

- 07:00-08:00: a glass of water (200 ml) and a spoon of psyllium bran.
- After 15 minutes, drink a mug of chamomile tea.

★ Breakfast

Almond milk and banana

🕐 Timeline: 08:00-09:00

One banana, cinnamon, almond milk 200 ml, 5 pieces of almonds, a spoon of rye/oat flakes.
Calories: **450 kcal**

How to prepare:

Mix everything in a blender or smoothie maker (it is called a smoothie shake).

Properties:

Cinnamon helps burn fat tissue. Bananas are an important source of potassium, a very important mineral. Oat flakes contain fibers which help regulate the intestinal transit.

Contraindications:

None

- Drink water after an hour.

★ Snack 1

A grapefruit

🕐　Time: 11:00

A grapefruit.
Calories: **100 kcal**

Properties:

It is a fruit low in calories, which helps burn fats and boosts the metabolism.

Contraindications:

None!

🥛　Drink 200 ml of marigold tea after an hour.

★ Lunch

Bone broth with vegetables

🕑　Timeline: 13:00 - 14:00:

Bone broth with vegetables: 2-3 pieces of bones, 2 carrots, 1 parsley, 1 parsnip, 1 kohlrabi. You will eat 150 ml.
Calories: **400 kcal**

How to prepare:

Let the chicken or cow bones simmer for 2-3 hours with a teaspoon of salt, add water on the way, then add the vegetables, boil them until they become soft, add parsley or lovage at the end, if preferred.

Properties:

It is a meal rich in proteins, vitamins and minerals.

Contraindications:

Egg may cause allergies

🥛　Drink 200 ml of water after an hour.

★ Snack 2

Almond milk

🕐　16:00

1 glass of almond milk (150 ml)
Calories: **200 kcal**

Properties:

It contains plant proteins, vitamins and minerals.

Contraindications:

None!

🥛　Drink water after 30 minutes.

★ Dinner

Mozzarella cheese

🕐 Timeline: 19:00 - 20:00:

70 g light mozzarella cheese, with oregano and a teaspoon of olive oil, 2 spoons of beans and a tomato.
Calories: **400 kcal**

How to prepare:

Cut the mozzarella, mix the ingredients, add chili flakes, salt and olive oil.

Properties:

It a delicious and light meal, it contains proteins, calcium potassium, manganese and vitamins. Fatty acids in the olive oil sustain blood vessels and heart.

Contraindications:

None!

🥛 Drink a glass of water after an hour.

🥛 Drink a glass of water with a teaspoon of flaxseed (previously hydrated in water for at least 4-5 hours) before bed.

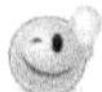

Now that you have finished your detox, please post your results on the group, in order to encourage other members, and tell us how you felt.
Leave your feedback on our Facebook page @NutriFitUp.

★ Bonus recipe ★

In case you have extra ingredients left, you can cook something tasty: cookies.

I want to show you the recipe Simona gave me. (Thank you once again, they are delicious!)

I put 3 ripe bananas, 200 g oats, I added all sorts of dried fruit, but also bananas – because they are very sweet. I let sit for about an hour.

Oat and bran biscuits: I put 3 bananas, 200 g oats, all sorts of dried fruit (no added sugar), a teaspoon of agave syrup (not mandatory), I mixed the ingredients and let sit for an hour covered with foil. I spread the dough and cut shapes, put them in the oven at 180 degrees, 20 minutes until golden.

Testimonials

Mariana 28, single, divorced:

"I lost 5 kg in one month, I always used to blame my work, I thought that is why I was gaining weight, but I discovered easy methods to prepare the food and I managed to adopt a healthy lifestyle, to exercise, to like my body and, what's more important, now that I am

healthy, I am no longer anemic. I didn't use to eat vegetables and fruit, I used to eat twice a day, and those times only bought food, I used to drink a glass of water at 14, compared to what my body needs, namely 3 liters. I will continue this lifestyle because now I feel extraodinary, thank you NutriFitUp, you are the answer I needed."

Denisa:

"Since I was born and up to 9 I had a normal weight; but I discovered sweets, fast-food and then my weight gain process began. I started eating frantically, schnitzels, meatballs, fries. At 14 I kept a hype diet, lost 10 kg then put 20 kg back on. Until 16 I gained and gained. Ever since I discovered nutrition and Detox NutriFitUp, combined with exercise, my habits have changed. I started loving sport and the fact that I feel good in my own skin. Thank you for all the support during these months."

Maria, 47, three kids, 2 miscarriages, surgeries...

"My life hasn't been quite easy, I realized that with the passing of time came the problems, I started eating chaotically, neglect myself, put family first, thinking it was good. Until one day when I fainted, exhausted to do all those things that I forgot to eat. The doctor told me if I want enjoy life with my children. I should make a change.

Then I understood that what I did was detrimental to my family. I've undergone treatment, but I started going to the gym, eat what NutriFitUp recommended, be strict with myself, but at the same time cherish myself more. It was interesting that I had the support of my family. I managed to lose weight and feel very good. According to the last visits at the doctor and the blood tests, I managed to get rid of blood pressure and cholesterol medicine and I think that as long as I carry on with a healthy lifestyle, I will not go through that again! After this detox I do not know what acid, stomach pain or constipation is."

Dorel:

"After this detox I can say that my life has changed, I eat healthy, I am no longer tired, and I have an incredible energy, I feel excellent, I will continue eating healthy!"

Dana:

"After this detox I did not feel bloated anymore, my transit changed. I go to the toilet daily and I love my new lifestyle, to which I never thought I would get accustomed."

Andreea:

"This detox made me understand how much harm I've done to my body: I drank liters of Coke and I could barely sleep because of the stomach pain, I did not eat as I wanted to lose weight and took painkillers by the handful. I have got rid of the stomach pain now, I gave up Coke and started exercising, running, living healthy!"

Dictionary

Detox - Metabolic action through which a toxic product is neutralized or it is transformed into a less toxic product.

A detox diet is necessary at least once every season. Detox can reduce the occurrence of health issues such as fatigue, low immunity, allergies, headaches, low concentration and skin itches.

Metabolism – All the synthesis complex processes, of assimilation (energy storage), degradation and disassembly (accompanied by energy release), suffered by substances in a living organism. ◊ Basal metabolism = the quantity of calories produced in an hour, while the body is at rest, reported to a square meter of the body surface.

Metabolism is made up of two processes: anabolism and catabolism. Anabolism represents all the chemical reactions of biosynthesis which need energy consumption. Catabolism represents all the reactions which lead to a degradation of the substances in the body, it generates a release of energy.

Cholesterol –Substance found, either free or combined, in fish oil, in the bile, blood, nervous tissue, egg yolk and which regulates the cells' permeability towards liquids.

High cholesterol is one of the main factors which determine the emergence of a disease, but we do need to acknowledge the fact that there are two types of cholesterol: good cholesterol HDL (high density lipoprotein) and bad cholesterol LDL (low-density lipoprotein).

LDL cholesterol (bad cholesterol) can attach to the blood vessels' walls. In time, this type of cholesterol, along with other substances, can clog the arteries. As such, the arteries inside the heart can be affected and blood clots can appear.

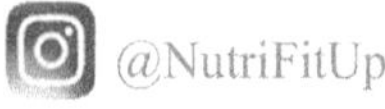

Visceral fat

> VISCERA All the organs inside the big cavities of bodies (Especially the abdominal cavity) in humans and animals; guts.

It is known as active and subcutaneous fat, the fat under the skin. It is hard to observe, as it surrounds organs such as liver, pancreas, and intestines.

Thin people can have high quantities of visceral fat, which is influenced by genetic factors negatively affecting health aspects.

Emollient 1-2 Medicine which softens hardened, inflamed or congested tissues 3 Substance used to finish textile products, to give them softness and shine.

Acts by softening scaly patches of the skin. Applied on the skin, these eliminate the surface harshness.

Vegetable oils which help the skin suppleness: Shea butter, Jojoba oil, grape seed oil, sesame oil, cocoa butter.

Antioxidant 1-2 Substance which prevents or delays the oxidation process.

Antioxidants are a complex of vitamins, minerals and specific enzymes which have the role to reduce the toxic effect of free radicals.

Free radicals are atoms or groups of atoms which, if not kept under control by antioxidants, might affect the immune system and can cause cardiac, pulmonary, mental disorders or cancer.

The most powerful antioxidants are: vitamin A, vitamin B complex (beta-carotene), vitamin C, vitamin E.

Triglycerides glycerin triester with fatty acids.

Triglycerides are fat substances which are synthesized by the human body from foods.

Triglycerides and cholesterol are interconnected, any person checking the value of their cholesterol most likely had their triglycerides checked too.

The increase in the level of triglycerides leads to weight gain and it also presents a risk of heart disease, as well as other disorders associated with an unhealthy lifestyle.

Additives 1 *regarding addition* 2 which is expressed through a physical measure whose value is expressed by algebraic sum 3. Substance which is added to a mineral oil or in preparing concrete to improve their properties.

An additive is a substance introduced in a mixture to give it characteristics, it is added in the processing or production process in order to enhance taste, flavor and looks and to extend shelf life.

Healthy lifestyle

Means healthy lifestyle and hydration, exercising, sport and rest. The diet is the key factor in a healthy lifestyle, as this must be based on fruit and vegetables, lean meat, whole meal cereals and healthy fats (Omega 3). Combined with movement and physical exercises, it helps maintaining a healthy figure. Stress is another factor which influences the functioning of the body. If the diet is balanced and combined with sport, then stress is reduced considerably.

Sedentary lifestyle

Is the lifestyle which does not involve moving around a lot or physical exercise. A sedentary lifestyle should be avoided as it can lead to several disorders (diabetes, obesity, heart problems). It is medically recommended to avoid sedentary habits.

CVA (cerebrovascular accident) is a medical emergency when the blood flow to the brain is interrupted.

The brain does not receive the necessary blood and oxygen quantity.

An unhealthy lifestyle can cause an CVA. In order to prevent such an accident, we must have a diet rich in fruits and vegetables, rest, and a healthy weight. We can also reduce the risk of having a stroke by quitting smoking and reducing the alcohol intake.

Nephrolithiasis

It is the term for kidney stones and it represents mineral bits at the kidney level, which can be eliminated through the urinary tract.
This disorder can appear due to insufficient hydration, or when the diet is poor in calcium or too rich in oxalates (chocolate).

Atherosclerosis

Chronic degenerative disease caused by fat and cholesterol masses on the internal wall of the arteries, determining their sclerosing.

The main causes of its emergence are type II diabetes, sedentary life, smoking, obesity, etc.
The lesions can cause a minor infarct, stroke, lower limbs arteritis, etc.

Intestinal barrier

It is made up of probiotics, which help the stomach's content not to reach the intestines.
Probiotics are different types of bacteria: some protect the intestines from harmful germs, some boost the immunity system, while others prevent digestive troubles. All these strengthen the intestinal barrier, which protects the whole body.

In the following pages you will discover the E-numbers tables, those Es that are very harmful and should be consumed as less often as possible, or not at all.

E numbers

	Index	Additive	Technological function	Toxicity level
1	E102	Tartrazine	Yellow artificial dye	Do not consume more than the recommended daily dose
2	E110	Sunset Yellow FCF; Orange Yellow S	Yellow dye	Frequent use is **NOT** recommended
3	E122	Azorubine; Carmoisine	Red artificial dye	Frequent use is NOT recommended
4	E123	Amaranth	Red artificial dye	NOT recommended
5	E124	Ponceau 4R; Cochineal Red A	Red artificial dye	NOT recommended
6	E127	Erythrosine	Red artificial dye	**NOT recommended**
7	E128	Red 2G	Red artificial dye	**Forbidden in the EU**
8	E129	Red Ac	Red artificial dye	Frequent use is NOT recommended
9	E131	Patent Blue V	Blue artificial dye	Frequent use is NOT recommended
10	E132	Indigotine; Indigo Carmine	Blue artificial dye	Frequent use is NOT recommended
11	E133	Brilliant Blue FCF	Blue artificial dye	Frequent use is NOT recommended
12	E142	Green S	Green dye	Frequent use is NOT recommended
13	E151	Brilliant Black BN; Black PN	Black dye	NOT recommended
14	E154	Brown FK	Brown dye	**NOT recommended**
15	E155	Brown HT	Brown dye	**NOT recommended**
16	E180	Lithol Rubine	Surface dye	Frequent use is NOT recommended
17	E210	Benzoic acid	Artificial preservative	Frequent use is NOT recommended, especially for sensitive people
18	E211	Sodium benzoate	Artificial preservative	Frequent use is NOT recommended, especially for sensitive people

	Index	Additive	Technological function	Toxicity level
19	E213	Calcium benzoate	Artificial preservative	Frequent use is NOT recommended, especially for sensitive people
20	E214	Ethyl p-hydroxybenzoate	Artificial preservative	Frequent use is NOT recommended, especially for sensitive people
21	E215	Sodium ethyl p-hydroxybenzoate	Artificial preservative	Frequent use is NOT recommended, especially for sensitive people
22	E216	Propylparaben	Artificial preservative	Frequent use is NOT recommended, especially for sensitive people
23	E217	Propil-p-Hydroxybenzoate	Artificial preservative	Frequent use is NOT recommended, especially for sensitive people
24	E218	Methyl p-hydroxybenzoate	Artificial preservative	Frequent use is NOT recommended, especially for sensitive people
25	E219	Sodium methyl p-hydroxybenzoate	Artificial preservative	Frequent use is NOT recommended, especially for sensitive people
26	E220	Sulphur dioxide	Preservative and antioxidant	Frequent use is NOT recommended, especially for sensitive people
27	E221	Sodium sulphite	Preservative and antioxidant	Frequent use is NOT recommended, especially for sensitive people
28	E222	Sodium hydrogen sulphite	Preservative and antioxidant	Frequent use is NOT recommended, especially for sensitive people

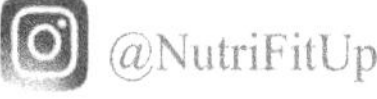

	Index	Additive	Technological function	Toxicity level
29	E223	Sodium metabisulphite	Preservative and antioxidant	Frequent use is NOT recommended, especially for sensitive people
30	E224	Potassium metabisulphite	Preservative and antioxidant	Frequent use is NOT recommended, especially for sensitive people
31	E226	Calcium sulphite	Preservative and antioxidant	Frequent use is NOT recommended, especially for sensitive people
32	E227	Calcium hydrogen sulphite	Preservative and antioxidant	Frequent use is NOT recommended, especially for sensitive people
33	E228	Potassium hydrogen sulphite	Preservative and antioxidant	Frequent use is NOT recommended, especially for sensitive people
34	E231	Phenylphenol	Surface preservative	**NOT recommended** fruit and shells
35	E232	Sodium orthophenyl phenol	Surface preservative	NOT recommended fruit and shells
36	E249	Potassium nitrite	Preservative, dye agent	Frequent use is NOT recommended, especially for sensitive people
37	E284	Boric acid	Preservative	Avoid use
38	E285	Sodium tetraborate; borax	Preservative	**NOT recommended**
39	E310	Propyl gallate	Antioxidant	Frequent use is NOT recommended
40	E312	Dodecyl gallate	Antioxidant	Frequent use is NOT recommended
41	E385	Calcium disodium ethylene diamine tetra-acetate	Preservative	NOT recommended

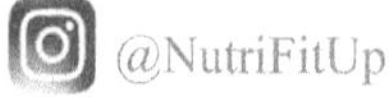

	Index	Additive	Technological function	Toxicity level
42	E1201	Polyvinyl-pyrrolidone	Thickening substance, humectant, stabilizer, ballast, texturing substance	Frequent use is NOT recommended
43	E1520	Propan-1,2-diol; propylene glycol	Humectant, solvent, oil based	NOT recommended

I would like to show you some natural E numbers, none of which is harmful. You can consume these without any problems:

- **Carotenoid or E160 – it is obtained from tomatoes and it is used to color foods. It is 1,000 times more preferred instead of carmine.**

- **E 162** – no harmful effects and it is obtained from beetroot. I use this ingredient to make ice cream for my daughters.

- **E 101, E 140,** vitamins equivalent to vitamin B12 and Vitamin E.

- **E 322** – known under the name of lecithin, it is obtained from soy. We still have a problem here, as there is synthetic lecithin and natural. Unfortunately, consumers cannot differentiate between the two.

If you liked *NutriFitUp* – 7-day Detox recommend it to other women in need!

Special Bonuses for you!

> Access:
> http://bit.ly/NutriFitUp-VIP
>
> and follow the steps
> (*prove you have bought this book*)
> **and become a member of NutriFitUp VIP
> community.**

Join the community of women who want, can and succeed!

Thank you for your involvement!

NutriFitUp Team

 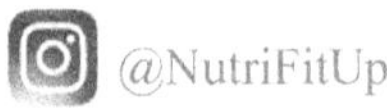

Bibliography

1. Dr. Phillis A. Balch. *Prescription for Nutritional Healing*, pg, 157, 159, 379. *Constipation*

2. Institute of Medicine, *Food and Nutrition Board. Dietary reference intakes for energy, carbohydrate, fiber, fat, fatty acids, cholesterol, protein, and amino acids (macronutrients).* Washington, DC: National Academy Press; 2005.

3. EFSA Panel on Dietetic Products, Nutrition, and Allergies (NDA); *Scientific, Opinion on Dietary Reference Values for fats, including saturated fatty acids, polyunsaturated fatty acids, monounsaturated fatty acids, trans fatty acids, and cholesterol.* EFSA Journal 2010

4. Siscovick DS & colab.: *Omega-3 polyunsaturated fatty acid (fish oil) supplementation and the prevention of clinical cardiovascular disease.* A science advisory from the American Heart Association. Circulation. http://circ.ahajournals.org/content/early/2017/03/13/CIR.0000000000000482

5. https://www.healthline.com/nutrition/11-proven-health-benefits-of-chia-seeds

6. https://www.healthline.com/health/psyllium-health-benefits#laxative

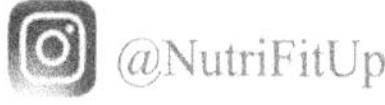

Ideas//observations//notes

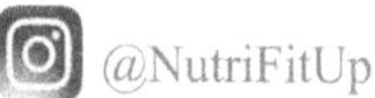

@NutriFitUp   @NutriFitUp

Ideas//observations//notes

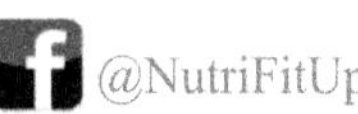

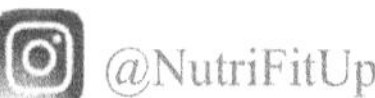

Ideas//observations//notes

 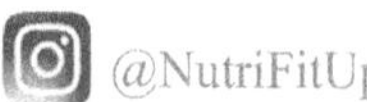 @NutriFitUp @NutriFitUp

Ideas//observations//notes

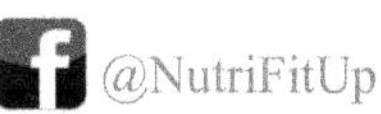

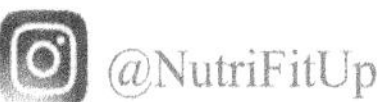

Ideas//observations//notes

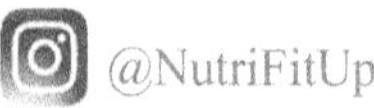

9 786069 500156